Tibetan Eye C

How to Improve Eyesight Using the Eye Chart, Keep Your Eyes Bright and Healthy

Aurelia Gold

DEDICATION

This book is dedicated to my lovely daughters Anna and Bella for their matchless effort and encouragement

TABLE OF CONTENT

CHAPTER 1

The History of the Tibetan Eye Chart - How It Came to Be and Its Significance Today

The Tibetan Eye Chart is a centuries-old instrument for improving eyesight and maintaining healthy eyes. Its origins can be traced back to Tibetan monks, who created the chart to aid in the improvement of their eyesight during lengthy periods of meditation. The chart is now widely used as a natural and successful means of enhancing vision without the use of corrective glasses or surgery.

The Tibetan Eye Chart is thought to have developed over a thousand years ago in the Tibetan Himalayas. The chart is made up of a series of sophisticated and geometric patterns, each of which is intended to stimulate different regions in the eyes. The chart was established by a lama, or spiritual instructor, who realized that his fellow monks' eyesight was deteriorating due to the extended periods of meditation they practiced.

The lama thought that, like any other part of the body, the eyes could be strengthened and exercised through specialized activities. He devised the Tibetan Eye Chart to assist his fellow monks in improving their vision and preventing additional injury. The chart was created to be used in conjunction with meditation and other practices to aid in the recovery and maintenance of the eyes' optimal health.

The Tibetan Eye Chart gained popularity outside of the monastery as time passed. People from all across Tibet and the rest of the world began to use the chart to improve their vision and keep their eyes healthy. The chart was especially popular among nomads who spent extended amounts of time in the harsh Tibetan climate, which might be very harmful to the eyes.

The Tibetan Eye Chart is now well-known around the world as a natural and effective means of enhancing eyesight. The chart is very popular among those who have myopia, hyperopia, astigmatism, or other visual difficulties. Its popularity has grown as more individuals seek natural and holistic approaches of health maintenance.

Despite its ancient origins, the Tibetan Eye Chart is still a useful tool for enhancing vision today. The chart is a monument to the Tibetan people's wisdom and expertise, who have long recognized the need of sustaining holistic health. Today, the chart is a helpful resource for those who want to improve their vision and keep their eyes healthy without the use of corrective lenses or surgery.

The Tibetan Eye Chart is notable not just for its efficiency as a tool for improving eyesight, but also for its spiritual and cultural value. The chart exemplifies the Tibetan people's rich and diversified culture, which has a long and storied history of spiritual and cultural rituals. The chart embodies the Tibetan people's wisdom and expertise, and serves as a reminder of their contributions to the world.

Finally, the Tibetan Eye Chart is an effective tool for increasing vision and preserving healthy eyes. Its ancient origins and spiritual importance attest to the Tibetan people's wisdom and expertise, and its popularity as a natural and holistic means of enhancing eyesight has only grown over time. The Tibetan Eye Chart is a vital resource for anyone looking to improve their eyesight and preserve healthy eyes as we continue to seek out natural and holistic techniques for managing our health.

Chapter 2

Understanding How the Tibetan Eye Chart Works - The Science Behind Its Effectiveness

The Tibetan Eye Chart is a centuries-old instrument for improving eyesight and maintaining healthy eyes. While the chart's origins are deep in tradition and spirituality, its success can be explained using scientific concepts. In this chapter, we'll look at the science behind the Tibetan Eye Chart and how it can help you see better.

The Tibetan Eye Chart stimulates specific areas in the eyes responsible for visual acuity. The chart is made up of a succession of complicated and geometric patterns, each of which is designed to target different parts of the eyes. The patterns are intended to exercise the muscles and nerves in the eyes, which can increase visual acuity and minimize eye strain.

The concept of eye muscle training is one of the major principles underlying the Tibetan Eye Chart's effectiveness. The muscles of the eyes, like any other muscle in the body, can be strengthened by particular exercises. The Tibetan Eye Chart is intended to target the muscles in the eyes, increasing their strength and flexibility over time.

The chart also helps with blood flow to the eyes. The chart can enhance blood flow to the eyes by stimulating certain areas of the eyes, which can supply critical nutrients and oxygen to the eyes. This can help to reduce eye strain and fatigue, which can be an issue for people who spend a lot of time gazing at screens or doing other visual chores.

The concept of eye relaxation is another aspect that contributes to the Tibetan Eye Chart's effectiveness. The chart is intended to aid in the relaxation of the eyes and the reduction of tension in the eye muscles. This is especially beneficial for those who have eye strain, which can cause discomfort and irritation in the eyes. The chart can alleviate pressure on the eyes and enhance general eye health by assisting them in relaxing.

The Tibetan Eye Chart, in addition to these concepts, aims to strengthen the coordination of the eyes and the brain. The chart is intended to activate both the left and right sides of the brain, improving coordination and balance between the two hemispheres. This can be especially beneficial for persons who struggle with depth perception and other visual tasks due to visual perception issues.

While the concepts underlying the Tibetan Eye Chart's efficacy are scientifically valid, it is crucial to highlight that the chart should not be utilized in place of professional medical care. Before using the chart, anyone with serious eye diseases or injuries should get medical attention.

Finally, the Tibetan Eye Chart is a useful tool for increasing vision and maintaining healthy eyes. Its effectiveness can be explained by scientific factors such as eye muscle training, increased blood flow to the eyes, ocular relaxation, and improved eye-brain coordination. While the chart should not be used in place of professional medical treatment, it can be a useful resource for those wishing to improve their vision and keep their eyes healthy.

Chapter 3

The Benefits of Using the Tibetan Eye Chart - Improving Eyesight Naturally

The Tibetan Eye Chart is a potent tool that has been used for millennia to improve vision and keep eyes healthy. The chart can assist to increase visual acuity and reduce eye strain by targeting specific parts of the eyes and exercising the muscles and nerves. In this chapter, we will look at the various advantages of adopting the Tibetan Eye Chart to naturally improve eyesight.

Enhancing Visual Acuity

One of the key advantages of adopting the Tibetan Eye Chart is that it improves visual acuity. The chart can assist to strengthen the muscles and nerves essential for clear vision by activating certain parts of the eyes. This is especially useful for people who have refractive problems like nearsightedness, farsightedness, or astigmatism.

Eye Strain Reduction

Many people suffer from eye strain and fatigue as a result of staring at displays or completing other visual chores for extended periods of time. The Tibetan Eye Chart can help reduce eye strain by exercising the eye muscles and encouraging eye relaxation. This can aid in reducing eye discomfort and fatigue, which can have a substantial impact on overall eye health.

Enhancing Eye Coordination

The Tibetan Eye Chart is intended to activate both the left and right sides of the brain, improving coordination and balance between the two hemispheres. This might be especially beneficial for those who struggle with depth perception or other visual perception issues.

Muscle Strengthening for the Eyes

The muscles of the eyes, like any other muscle in the body, can be strengthened by particular exercises. The Tibetan Eye Chart is intended to target the muscles in the eyes, increasing their strength and flexibility over time. This can lessen the likelihood of eye injuries and enhance general eye health.

Boosting Blood Flow to the Eyes

The Tibetan Eye Chart can enhance blood flow to the eyes by stimulating certain parts of the eyes. This can assist to lessen eye strain and exhaustion by providing important nutrients and oxygen to the eyes. Improved blood flow can also aid in the prevention of eye diseases such as glaucoma and cataracts.

Increasing Eye Relaxation

The Tibetan Eye Chart is intended to induce eye relaxation, which can be especially beneficial for those who suffer from eye strain and weariness. The chart helps relieve stress in the eye muscles and enhance general eye health by encouraging relaxation.

Enhancing Overall Eye Health

The Tibetan Eye Chart has been shown to improve general eye health. The chart can assist to maintain healthy eyes and reduce the risk of eye illnesses and injuries by enhancing visual acuity, lowering eye strain, strengthening eye muscles, increasing blood flow to the eyes, promoting eye relaxation, and improving eye coordination.

To summarize, the Tibetan Eye Chart is a wonderful tool for organically enhancing eyesight. The chart can assist to improve visual acuity, reduce eye strain, strengthen eye muscles, increase blood flow to the eyes, promote eye relaxation, and improve general eye health by targeting particular areas of the eyes and exercising the muscles and nerves. While the chart should not be used in place of professional medical treatment, it can be a useful resource for people wishing to naturally maintain healthy eyes and improve their vision.

Chapter 4

Preparing to Use the Tibetan Eye Chart - Getting Started with the Chart

Before you start using the Tibetan Eye Chart, take some time to prepare and make sure you have everything you need to get the most out of it. In this chapter, we'll go through how to get ready to utilize the Tibetan Eye Chart and offer some pointers on how to get started.

Choosing an Appropriate Location

The first step in getting ready to utilize the Tibetan Eye Chart is deciding on an appropriate location. You should choose a peaceful and comfortable location where you can sit or stand for an extended period of time. The space should be well-lit and free of distractions like television, music, or other visual stimulation.

Gathering the Required Materials

You will need a copy of the Tibetan Eye Chart and a surface to place it on, such as a table or desk, to utilize it. You should also have a pen or pencil on hand to keep track of your development over time. It's also a good idea to have a comfy chair or cushion to sit on.

The Chart's Interpretation

Before you start using the Tibetan Eye Chart, you should understand how it works and what each symbol means. Spend some time studying the chart and becoming acquainted with the symbols and their meanings.

Techniques for Relaxation

It is critical to remain comfortable and attentive in order to get the most out of the Tibetan Eye Chart. Begin by practicing relaxation techniques like deep breathing or meditation. These approaches can aid in the reduction of stress and tension in the body, which can enhance your entire experience with the chart.

Exercises for the Eyes

It is recommended that you conduct some simple eye exercises before utilizing the Tibetan Eye Chart to warm up the muscles and nerves in your eyes. These exercises can help to prepare your eyes for the more difficult tasks on the chart. ocular rotations, blinking exercises, and palming are all examples of ocular exercises.

Time Administration

Using the Tibetan Eye Chart necessitates a major time commitment, and it is critical to schedule enough time each day to perform the exercises. Start with small sessions of 10-15 minutes and progressively increase the duration as you become more familiar with the chart.

Consistency

When utilizing the Tibetan Eye Chart, consistency is essential. To get the most out of the chart, it must be used on a regular and consistent basis. Make it a part of your regular routine to do your eye exercises at a specific time each day.

Persistence and patience

It takes time and perseverance to improve your eyesight with the Tibetan Eye Chart. You may not see immediate results, but with perseverance and determination, you will begin to notice improvements over time. It is critical to remain patient and consistent in your efforts, as well as committed to using the chart on a regular basis.

Finally, preparing to use the Tibetan Eye Chart is a vital step toward naturally improving your eyesight. You can get the most out of the chart and achieve significant improvements in your vision by selecting a suitable location, gathering the necessary materials, understanding the chart, practicing relaxation techniques and eye exercises, managing your time effectively, being consistent, and remaining patient and persistent. The Tibetan Eye Chart, with dedication and commitment, can be a great tool for preserving healthy eyes and increasing your general quality of life.

Chapter 5

Using the Tibetan Eye Chart - Proper Techniques and Best Practices

Now that you've prepared to use the Tibetan Eye Chart, it's time to delve into the procedures and best practices for doing so. In this chapter, we'll go through how to use the chart correctly and give you some pointers on how to achieve the greatest results.

Beginning with the Fundamental Symbols

When first using the Tibetan Eye Chart, it is recommended that you start with the basic symbols at the top of the chart. These symbols are easier to focus on and will prepare your eyes for the more complex ones.

Techniques for Concentration

It is critical to apply proper focusing skills when utilizing the Tibetan Eye Chart. Focusing on one sign at a time, using your peripheral vision to take in the surrounding symbols, and blinking between symbols to avoid eye strain are all examples of this.

Lighting

When using the Tibetan Eye Chart, proper illumination is crucial. The room should be well-lit, and the chart should be free of glare and reflections. It's also a good idea to avoid staring straight at bright lights, which can cause eye strain.

Distance

It is critical to keep the right distance from the Tibetan Eye Chart when using it. The chart should be put at a reasonable distance from you so that you can focus on the symbols without straining your eyes.

Duration

The length of your Tibetan Eye Chart eye exercises will vary based on your level of experience and comfort. Start with shorter sessions of 10-15 minutes and progressively expand the duration as you become more familiar with the chart.

Taking a Break

It is critical to rest your eyes after working with the Tibetan Eye Chart. Close your eyes or look aside from the chart for a few minutes to do this. This will allow your eyes to relax and heal before you begin your next session.

Monitoring Progress

Using the Tibetan Eye Chart to track your progress is a crucial aspect of the process. You can achieve this by keeping track of the symbols you can focus on and the length of your sessions. This will allow you to track your progress over time and alter your exercises as needed.

Including the Chart in Your Routine

It is critical to include the Tibetan Eye Chart into your daily practice in order to get the most out of it. Setting out a specified time each day for eye exercises or combining the exercises into other activities, such as reading or watching television, may be helpful.

Seeking Professional Help

While the Tibetan Eye Chart can be an effective tool for naturally improving your eyesight, it is critical to seek expert guidance if you have any concerns about your vision. Your eye doctor can give you vital information and direction on how to use the chart successfully and securely.

To summarize, using the Tibetan Eye Chart involves proper approaches and best practices in order to achieve the greatest outcomes. You can achieve significant improvements in your vision and maintain healthy eyes by beginning with the basic symbols, using proper focusing techniques, ensuring proper lighting and distance, managing your duration and rest periods, tracking your progress, incorporating the chart into your routine, and seeking professional advice when necessary. The Tibetan Eye Chart, with dedication and commitment, can be a helpful tool for improving your entire quality of life.

Chapter 6

Eye Exercises to Supplement the Tibetan Eye Chart - Additional Methods to Improve Eyesight

While the Tibetan Eye Chart is an effective tool for naturally increasing eyesight, there are other eye exercises that can supplement its use and bring even more benefits for your vision. In this chapter, we'll look at some of these exercises and how they can be combined with the Tibetan Eye Chart.

Palming

Palming is a simple and efficient eye relaxation and strain reduction technique. To begin, sit in a comfortable position and lay your palms over your eyes, fingers interlocking at the brow.

Close your eyes and concentrate on the darkness, as if you are completely enveloped in it. Perform this exercise for a few minutes every time your eyes become weary or strained.

Eye Movements

Eye rotations can help to enhance your eyes' flexibility and range of motion, which can improve your overall vision. Sit in a comfortable position and look straight ahead to do this exercise. Slowly spin your eyeballs clockwise for a few rotations, then counterclockwise, without moving your head. To increase your eye mobility, perform this exercise for a few minutes each day.

Blinking

Blinking is a simple and efficient practice for enhancing attention and reducing eye strain. Sit in a comfortable position and blink your eyes quickly for a few seconds, then close them and relax them for a few seconds. Repeat for a few minutes to relieve eye strain and enhance focus.

Close-up Focus

Near-far focus exercises can help to increase your eyes' capacity to adjust to varied distances, hence improving your overall vision. Sit in a comfortable position and place your thumb about 10 inches away from your face to perform this exercise. Focus on your thumb for a few seconds, then change your attention to a distant object. For a few minutes, alternate your focus between your thumb and the distant object to strengthen your near-far vision.

Visualizing

Visualization exercises can help you enhance your capacity to envision and visualize items in your mind, which can help you see better overall. To begin, sit in a comfortable position and visualize a basic object in your mind, such as a ball or a cube. Try to imagine the thing as precisely as possible, including its size, form, and color. To strengthen your visualization skills and general vision, spend a few minutes each day imagining items.

Breathing

Breathing exercises can help reduce stress and tension in the eyes, improving overall eyesight. Sit in a comfortable position and take slow, deep breaths, concentrating on the sensation of air moving in and out of your body. Imagine that you are breathing in fresh, healing air that is feeding your eyes as you breathe. To alleviate stress and tension in the eyes, perform this exercise for a few minutes each day.

Finally, while the Tibetan Eye Chart is a wonderful tool for naturally increasing eyesight, there are other activities that can supplement its use and bring even more benefits for your vision. You can improve your general eye health and vision by including activities such as palming, eye rotations, blinking, near-far concentration, visualizing, and breathing into your daily routine. These exercises can be a beneficial addition to your eye care routine and help you attain maximum eye health with effort and commitment.

Chapter 7

Nutrition and Eye Health - How Diet Affects Eyesight and How to Eat for Optimal Eye Health

Diet is extremely important in preserving healthy eyesight. Foods include nutrients that are necessary for good eye health. In this chapter, we will look at the relationship between diet and eye health and offer advice on how to eat for best eye health.

Essential nutrients for vision health

Several nutrients are required for optimal eye health, including:

Vitamin A: This nutrient is necessary for good eye health. Foods high in vitamin A include liver, sweet potatoes, carrots, and spinach.

Vitamin C is a potent antioxidant that can help protect the eyes from harm. It can be found in citrus fruits, bell peppers, and broccoli.

Vitamin E: An antioxidant, this nutrient can help protect the eyes from harm. It can be found in almonds, sunflower seeds, and spinach.

Zinc: Zinc is required for healthy vision and can be found in foods such as oysters, steak, and pumpkin seeds.

Omega-3 fatty acids: Found in foods such as salmon, sardines, and walnuts, these fatty acids are vital for sustaining healthy vision.

Foods that are good for your eyes

Several foods can help with eye health, including:

Leafy green vegetables, such as spinach, kale, and collard greens, are high in lutein and zeaxanthin, which can help protect the eyes.

Carrots are high in beta-carotene, which the body converts into vitamin A.

Citrus fruits, such as oranges and grapefruits, are high in vitamin C and can help protect the eyes from harm.

Eggs are high in lutein and zeaxanthin, both of which can help protect the eyes from harm.

Nuts and seeds: Nuts and seeds high in vitamin E and zinc include almonds, sunflower seeds, and chia seeds.

Fish: Fatty fish like salmon and sardines are high in omega-3 fatty acids, which can help keep your eyesight healthy.

Dietary Guidelines for Good Eye Health

Consider the following guidelines for eating for best eye health:

Consume a well-balanced diet rich in fruits, vegetables, whole grains, lean proteins, and healthy fats.

Include foods high in eye-healthy minerals such as vitamin A, vitamin C, vitamin E, zinc, and omega-3 fatty acids.

Consume fewer processed and fried foods, which are heavy in harmful fats and sodium.

Instead of frying, choose healthy cooking methods such as grilling, baking, or steaming.

Avoid smoking since it increases the risk of eye problems including macular degeneration.

Drink plenty of water throughout the day to stay hydrated.

Finally, food is important in preserving healthy eyesight. You may help protect your eyes from damage and maintain optimal eye health by include foods rich in nutrients needed for eye health in your diet, such as leafy green vegetables, citrus fruits, eggs, nuts, seeds, and seafood. You may enhance your general eye health and keep clear and healthy vision for years to come by eating a balanced and healthy diet, getting regular eye exams, and using the Tibetan Eye Chart and eye exercises.

Chapter 8

Lifestyle Changes to Improve Eyesight - Tips for Adjusting Habits to Promote Healthy Vision

There are various lifestyle adjustments you may do to promote good vision, in addition to using the Tibetan Eye Chart, eye exercises, and eating a nutritious food. In this chapter, we'll look at some strategies for changing your behaviors to improve your vision.

Take a break from your screens.

Many of us spend a lot of time staring at screens, whether they be on our computers, phones, or televisions. This can result in eye strain, fatigue, and possibly long-term vision difficulties. It is critical to take breaks from screens throughout the day to avoid this. Follow the 20-20-20 rule: take a 20-second break every 20 minutes and look at something 20 feet away. This can aid in the reduction of eye strain and fatigue.

Make changes to your lighting.

Your eyesight might also be affected by the lighting in your environment. Eye strain and weariness can be caused by too much or too little light. To avoid this, make sure your surroundings are well-lit. When working on a computer or reading, use a task light and avoid working in dimly lit places. Adjust the brightness of your screens as well to avoid eye strain.

Get enough rest.

Sleeping enough is essential for general health, including eye health. Sleep deprivation can result in eye strain, dry eyes, and other vision issues. To promote healthy vision, aim for 7-8 hours of sleep per night.

Exercise on a regular basis.

Regular exercise is not only beneficial to general health, but it can also aid in the promotion of healthy vision. Exercise helps enhance blood flow to the eyes and lower the risk of vision issues like glaucoma and age-related macular degeneration. Aim for 30 minutes of moderate exercise every day, such as walking, running, or swimming.

Wear safety glasses.

Wear protective eyewear if you participate in activities that could result in eye injury, such as sports or working with power tools. This can aid in the prevention of eye injuries and the promotion of healthy vision.

Stop smoking

Smoking is bad for your whole health, especially your eyes. It has been linked to an increased risk of eye illnesses such as cataracts and age-related macular degeneration. If you smoke, you should think about stopping to promote healthy vision.

Maintain good hygiene.

Good cleanliness is essential for preventing eye infections and other vision disorders. Regularly wash your hands, especially before touching your eyes or putting on contact lenses.

Additionally, to avoid infections, replace your contact lenses as directed.

Finally, there are a number of lifestyle adjustments you may undertake to enhance healthy eyesight. Taking breaks from screens, adjusting your lighting, getting enough sleep, exercising regularly, wearing protective eyewear, quitting smoking, and practicing excellent hygiene are all things that can help support healthy vision and lower the risk of visual disorders. You can enhance your general eye health and preserve clear and healthy vision for years to come by adopting these guidelines into your daily routine, along with the usage of the Tibetan Eye Chart, eye exercises, and a balanced diet.

Chapter 9

Success Stories: Real-Life Accounts of People Who Have Improved Their Eyesight with the Tibetan Eye Chart

For generations, the Tibetan Eye Chart has been utilized as a natural means of enhancing eyesight. While some may be skeptical of its efficacy, there have been numerous success stories from people who have used the chart to enhance their vision. In this chapter, we'll look at some real-life examples of people who have improved their vision using the Tibetan Eye Chart.

The Story of John

John had worn glasses for the most of his life and had grown tired of the trouble they created. After reading about the Tibetan Eye Chart's benefits online, he decided to give it a try. He employed the chart for several weeks, following the procedures and practices advised. After a few weeks, he found that his vision had greatly improved. For the first time in years, he could read without glasses, and his eyes were no longer strained or tired. He kept using the chart and ultimately quit wearing glasses altogether.

Maria's Experience

Maria had glaucoma and had been informed by her doctor that she would soon lose her vision. She chose to try the Tibetan Eye Chart as a natural way to improve her vision and delay the advancement of her glaucoma. She utilized the chart every day for several months, following the strategies and procedures advised. When she returned to her doctor for a check-up, he was surprised to notice that her vision had greatly improved. Her glaucoma had also advanced slower than expected. Maria maintains her improved vision by continuing to utilize the Tibetan Eye Chart as part of her daily routine.

Sarah's Experience

Sarah had been suffering from eye strain and headaches as a result of working long hours in front of a computer screen. To alleviate her discomfort, she decided to try the Tibetan Eye Chart. She utilized the chart for several weeks, following the approaches and procedures advised. After a few weeks, she realized that her eyes were no longer strained or fatigued, and her headaches were gone. She continued to utilize the chart on a daily basis and has been able to work comfortably in front of a computer screen without suffering any more symptoms.

Tom's Experience

Tom had age-related macular degeneration, which had resulted in substantial visual loss in his right eye. He chose to use the Tibetan Eye Chart to improve his vision naturally. He utilized the chart every day for several months, following the approaches and procedures advised. After a few months, he discovered that his vision in his right eye had greatly improved. He continued to utilize the chart on a regular basis and was able to keep his improved vision.

These are just a few of the numerous success stories from people who utilized the Tibetan

Eye Chart to improve their vision. While each person's experience will vary, it is obvious that the chart can be an effective natural way for increasing vision. You, too, can benefit from enhanced vision by following the recommended techniques and practices and incorporating the chart into your daily routine.

Printed in Great Britain
by Amazon